Making Wellness Work

Practical tools and tips for lifetime success

By: Heather Preston-Weeks MA, CHES, ACSM-CPT,CHWC

Dedicated to all of my former and future clients who make an effort each day to change their lives for the better. You are worth it!

Chapters

Chapter 1

Why are you here?

The foundation of behavior change

"Whether you think you can or you can't, you will always be right." Profound words from the founder of our modern automobile Mr. Henry Ford; and nothing could be more true, which is why I want to begin by discussing the reasons that you have chosen to begin (or return to) your wellness journey by purchasing this book. What is it that has brought you here for what might be the first or the 50th time in your life? What do you want to accomplish within the next 8 chapters that you were not able to before? These questions are important ones to answer prior to beginning any of the exercises that are within these pages; for understanding the "why" of what brought you here will lay the foundation for what is yet to come. So, let's take a few minutes to begin this process and discuss where behavior change starts. Quite simply, behavior change begins within all of us;

our mindset. Our intentions regarding what we should and should not be doing with our health, or what we want for our life, begins with our thoughts on the subject. Do we really want it?

If you really want something, do you usually get it? Think about the times in your life when you wanted a particular job, to get into a certain college, or secure the interests of a certain person; you probably succeeded when the desire was greatest. When you really want something, your thoughts, words, and actions all reflect the positive future that you are seeking. That laser focus you have about your future is what gets you there! This is what it takes for true behavior change. The very first agenda item is that you must really WANT to change. If you have this desire then you will be working successfully with the first tool necessary to reach your wellness goals.

Most of us want quick fixes when we seek change in our health, weight, looks, or social status. We want it NOW! In the short term, we may feel a false sense of pleasure from attaining a quick fix goal, but in the long run we jeopardize our confidence more and more each time the change does not last. This is what creates that mindset of "I can never do it." and "I always fail so why try again?". Wouldn't you like to break that cycle once and for all and learn how to keep things simple so that change can last a lifetime? Isn't it time to sort through the bewildering array of health information, products, and services that seem to do the trick but never really last? Now is the time to take charge of your life and begin to learn new skills, new ways of thinking, and gather more tools to change your behavior for once and for all!

It does not matter if your goal is to lose weight, improve your eating habits, find time to exercise, improve your self-esteem, find a new career, quit smoking, or any combination of these; behavior change begins with your *idea* about things and the *action* that develops from it.

Change of any kind *can* and *will* take place if you use the advice and tools that have been presented and tested in multiple health behavior theories; the theories that will be touched upon throughout this book. So, take a deep breath, sit back, and begin to focus on what you truly want to achieve in this life and I guarantee you have the ability to get there. Follow me and I will show you the way. Let's get started!

Chapter 2

Getting it right this time:

Eliminating the "quick fix" strategy

Let's get one thing straight; change will only occur if it is **your** idea, not someone else's. Ask yourself what it is that you really want to accomplish; what is your mind-set regarding this issue, positive or negative? Is this something that *you* really want? If it is positive and it is something that you really want, chances are changes WILL happen. Problems arise when someone is being told they *have* to do something. When they embark on behavior change for the wrong reasons, plans are certain to fall apart. Has anyone ever told you that you *have* to quit smoking, or you *should* lose some weight? Chances are when you tried to appease these individuals you did not make permanent changes in your life and became very frustrated in the process. Sound familiar?

The fact is, the first rule of behavior change is that the individual must WANT to make the change themselves, or else it is never going to work. When you really want something your thoughts, words, and actions reflect upon the changes you are seeking and you surround yourself with positive affirmations of what is to come. The saying "If you see it you can be it." is really true. Actually WANTING to make a change is the very first step in behavior modification. So ask yourself, are you ready for change right now? Be honest. What health behaviors would you like to improve upon? What do you want to be doing differently one year from now? Think about this, and begin to create a positive image of what the future "you" will look like and feel like.

Creating this Wellness Vision is the first step you can take to begin creating a new you and to change negative behaviors.

We will talk more about planning this vision a little later, but keep it on the back burner as we continue our conversation about *why* and *how* people change. This is the beginning of Behavior Theory 101. Well, not really. I am not going to go too deep with any of these theories and I don't expect you to be as enamored of them as I was during my graduate studies, but I do think it is important to give you a brief summary of the theories that are primarily used in most behavior modification systems. Let's start with the one that really gives us an accurate picture of why people either change, or don't; The Health Belief Model.

This was one of the first theories developed exclusively for health behavior, way back in the 1950's. It originated from the works of a few social psychologists who worked in the public health services. During this time there were many public health awareness campaigns for various diseases that were occurring across the country. One such campaign was sending mobile chest x-ray units to neighborhoods to conduct free tuberculosis screenings for everyone. Now, in my opinion I have a saying that if it is free it's for me, but not so with these folks! You see, very few people took advantage of this free service; they simply were not using the testing machines and the social psychologists wondered why.

To help them explain this phenomenon and to help recruit more "takers" the group looked into some existing theories of the time and then ultimately developed their own; The Health Belief Model. After doing their research, what they found was that when it comes to a health behavior, a person first needs to feel like they are at risk. If they don't, then they are less likely to care about it or do any sort of preventative maintenance. The second finding was that the person also has to have some sort of perceived severity of the issue. One person might have thought that TB was a death sentence while another person may have thought it was no big deal. Do you see where I am going with this? A person needs to *believe* that a health issue is a big deal and that they are *susceptible* in order for them to do anything about it. It needs to be seen as a threat in order for a person to feel compelled to take action.

So, these gentlemen figured this out, and this explained why people were not utilizing the free mobile x-ray units; they didn't think TB was going to affect them, so why get a chest x-ray? Hence, the Health Belief Model. I just love that story! It reminds me of the complex thought processes of an individual that must be sifted through in order to find out if a person is even *ready* for behavior change. We are indeed complex creatures! Perhaps you find yourself in this same frame of mind; you may not think there are any issues, so why do anything about it? You may not think you have a problem with smoking, stress, or with overeating, so there is really nothing to work on, right? But on the other hand, I would bet a lot of money that if you picked up this book and are still reading it, you really *do* believe that there is something you want to change.

That is why you are here.

So, you have now crossed over the bridge of believing that there is a health issue at hand and now you want to know how to change it. Well, let's talk about one more health behavior theory before we get into all of our tools and tactics. The most utilized and most important theory in my opinion is the Transtheorectical Model; referred to as the Stages of Change.

The Stages of Change Model was developed in the late 1970s by Dr. James Prochaska who reviewed various theories behind psychotherapy. In the process, he laid the foundation for this model. He found that there were certain commonalities in the process of changing behaviors within various therapies, which begins with a person's attitude towards change and then develops into stages of readiness.

The major premise of stage theory is that behavior change takes place over time and has to do with a person's psychological state as well as personality traits. When a person begins to consider a behavior change they move through five distinct stages during the process. These stages are: Precontemplation, Contemplation, Preparation, Action, and Maintenance. Understanding what each of these stages signifies will not only help you understand the behavior change process from start to finish, but can help you decide what stage you're currently in; this can help an individual work on his/her needs during that particular time in order to gradually move to the next stage as they get closer and closer to permanent change.

Now, stay with me here. We only have a few more items to discuss until you are all done with Behavior Change 101; I promise! It's important to understand the definition of each stage and some tools to carry you through each phase so you have more tricks up your sleeve. Just give me a few more paragraphs and you will soon be a Transtheorectical Model expert!

Stage One is the **Precontemplation** Stage. In this stage, the person is not even thinking about change, nor is it on their radar. They are not planning to make any behavior changes in the near future because they don't think they need to. Think of the people from the Health Belief Model story; they did not think they were at risk, so TB testing was not something they even considered.

Here, we need to just let people try to figure it out by giving them information (when accepted) and try not to be too pushy. Public service messages, pamphlets, and simply being around people who are in a healthier state of mind are all ways that a Precontemplater can move to the next stage.

Stage Two is **Contemplation**. A person in this stage is beginning to consider the benefits of changing their behavior and starting to put ideas on the backburner. They have no immediate plans to change, but may do so within the next 6 months. Information continues to be extremely important during this stage and people may ask for more of it by inquiring about gym memberships, talking to their doctor, or looking up specifics on the internet.

They are in, what I like to call, the perusal state; just dipping their toe in and deciding if and when they want to take the plunge.

When a person does decide to jump in, they are in the **Preparation** Stage of behavior change. This is when they are planning to actually make a change within the next month; they purchase the gym membership, buy new running shoes, get the nicotine replacement therapy, create space in their schedule for exercise, purchase new cookbooks, etc, etc. etc. At this point, you are at the starting line just waiting for the gun to go off; you are finally ready to make a change!

Now, the gun has gone off and you push off the starting block taking your first few steps towards the future you.

You are now in the **Action** Stage of this model; a time when you are actively participating in the new behavior from the very first day up to 6 months. A person in this stage needs to have continuous support and encouragement from themselves as well as those around them. They need to reward themselves for the changes they are making as they move along in the process.

After this, we consider the person to be in the **Maintenance** Stage. This final stage is where a person is maintaining their new behaviors for a long period of time, after the 6 month mark. Take heed at this point, for here is where you need everything in your bag of tricks! It is common for people to lose steam over time, fall off the wagon, hit a plateau, or become bored after many months of change.

New workouts, different recipes, alternate schedules, varying activities, or new social outlets are all things that should be considered to continue to keep the spice in your new routine.

To help you prepare for this stage, think about all possible road blocks you may encounter when you first embark in the process and come up with a plan of action with a list of potential fixes so that you don't fall back into old habits as you continue to maintain the new you. The Maintenance Stage is the pinnacle of your success; it shows you that you can do it, but it is also the place where people grow complacent and stagnate, so keep this in mind as you set out on your journey.

One last thing to keep in mind is that the process of change is not linear; we do not graduate from one stage and then go to the next without looking back.

Not so! The Stage Model is more like a ladder where you steadily move up each rung, but then may have a slight slip and need to step back down to a lower elevation once more. A person in the Action Stage might stay there for a month or so, but then find themselves struggling or getting discouraged, and move back into the Contemplation Stage ("Maybe I'll try this again in a few months when things aren't so hectic.") Then New Year rolls around and they find themselves back in the Preparation Stage, then finally in the action stage once more to try to change yet again. Sound familiar?

I bet you didn't know you were moving up and down the ladder of the Stages of Change all these years!

Now that you have a little knowledge about the main points of behavior theory, it will be easier to distinguish where you are in the process of change.

Perhaps *this* time it will be a little easier for you.

This time change will happen! No more quick fixes.

Chapter 3

Let's get started!

Beginning your journey towards wellness goals

Okay, so how do you get it right this time? How do you erase the past and forget about quick-fix plans? I will tell you all that and more. First and foremost, you use the health behavior theories to your advantage by understanding yourself, and then making a purposeful statement about the "future you"; see yourself in a vision of the future. We then create baby steps working towards this vision by establishing clear goals to help get you there. Your first step is creating your vision of where and how you want to be, your Wellness Vision! Creating a vision provides the framework to help you achieve optimal health and wellness. It is a statement written in the present tense, as if it is already happening to you; this way you can actually begin to live your life in that direction simply by reading your statement and planting that seed in your mind!

A Wellness Vision is not simply thinking about where you *hope* you will be 6-12 months from now; it is a powerful, positive statement indicting what you *will* be doing by that time. If you solely rely on motivation for behavior change you will find yourself giving up and giving in to what feels comfortable and familiar. With a clear plan of action you will know what to do to achieve your desired outcomes and make this vision a reality. Creating a Wellness Vision statement is your starting point for change.

Now, there are several different ways of doing this, but my favorite is in paragraph form. This gives you a "short story" version of the new you and allows you to be creative in the process. Here is an example:

"I am a lean, mean, fitness machine! I have been doing 3-4 kickboxing workouts every week at the gym and also walk during my lunch break at work. Doing this has helped me to lose 20 pounds and become the toned and defined person I knew was hiding all these years. My eating habits are better as well; I have my fruit and veggie protein shakes every morning and always pack healthy snacks for work. I am so much more organized than I used to be, and this has really helped with the process! I like the way I look and love the abundant amount of energy I have. My biggest supporters are my husband and kids, and they are so proud of me! I know that I am on the right path and I will continue to stay on it for a lifetime. I feel awesome!"

Wow, doesn't that feel great! Yes, I said *feel.* This statement is truly written as if these changes have already occurred and this person is living her ultimate life. You can sense this and feel what that must be like when reading her Wellness Vision. This is what I mean by writing in the present tense, as if these changes that you desire have already occurred. By doing this you are creating a very powerful tool for change. By reading your positive, in the now, Wellness Vision over and over again you are literally *seeing it* so you can *be it*! The brain is a marvelous thing; once you set your mind in a certain direction and see where you want to be, you will start living in that direction before you even realize it! Pretty neat, huh? Give it a try yourself, and don't worry if you're not a New York Times best- selling author; just keep the statements positive and in the present.

Stop here and take some time to develop your vision, as this is the very first step towards behavior change. Don't worry, I will still be waiting here when you return, and then we can go onto the next step in the process; taking baby steps. Here are a few phrases to get you started. Simply complete the sentences with words relating to what you need and desire and then take those to form a complete wellness paragraph that tells your story. Give it a try!

By this time next year I am…. I will be…

I am able to do this because I…..

The strengths that I draw upon to make these things happen are…

The people and resources that I have to help me are…

I am confident that I can continue with these habits because…

Make sure to end your paragraph with a positive statement about how all of this makes you feel, such as "Now that I have a slimmer figure and am keeping my body fueled with nutritious foods, I feel amazing!"

- Now it's your turn! Stop now and begin to write your Wellness Vision. Take some time to really think about *what* you want and *how* you will be in the future. Come back when you have a rough draft, and we will work on it and tweak it more as we move through this process.

Chapter 4

Key concepts of goal setting reviewed

Case Study

Okay, so now that you have a clear idea of where you want to be 6 months to a year from now, and have written a positive present-tense statement in paragraph form, (remember, no "I would like to be…" statements) you are now ready to break that down into more manageable steps. Let's begin to take those baby steps towards your ultimate self! We will begin with a medium-term goal set out at about 3 months. With this, your goal is short enough to present a sense of urgency for you so that you are more likely to take the weekly steps required to get to this point. It is important to break down your Wellness Vision to a more manageable chunk for this marker. Try extracting a few of the main themes from your long-term vision and include them in 2 or 3 specific goals. What *will you* be doing in 3-months' time? Ask yourself what specific behaviors you will be doing *consistently* 3 months from now. If we take the example from the previous chapter, this person's 3-Month Goals might sound something like this:

In three months' time I am doing 2 kickboxing classes per week consistently. I am drinking a veggie protein shake 3 mornings before I go to work. I spend 10 minutes two evenings per week getting my snack bags ready to take to work the next day.

These goals are simply a smaller piece of the larger puzzle, but certainly a major accomplishment and something to strive for in the nearer-term. Take a moment right now to extract a few items from your Wellness Vision and create your 3-Month Goal.

- Stop here and take a few moments to write 3 or 4 sentences that say what you will be doing by the 3-month mark. Don't rush this process of goal setting; take your time.

Finally, setting Weekly Goals is the last step in breaking down your vision into more palatable bites. Setting clear goals each week will be a specific plan of action (with some urgency) that will take you towards your 3-Month Goal and finally the Wellness Vision.

Weekly Goals also are very important in building up your self-efficacy which ultimately is what is going to keep you on track while you are making your way to the more long-term goals. How do we do this? We write clear Weekly Goals by using the SMART method; effective behavioral goals are Specific, Measurable, Action-based, Realistic, and Time-lined. For instance, walking two nights a week is specific, measurable, and action-based, doing it for 30 minutes is time-lined, and overall it is realistic. Goals should be written in a confident voice as with the previous goal- setting strategies, and they should push you just a bit beyond your comfort zone.

Setting appropriate goals is very important for you to gain self-confidence and self-efficacy. This is the backbone of the goal-setting process and is why it is so important to keep your goals "doable".

Think about this; if goals are too easy you really will not have to work hard to achieve them and will not feel accomplished when you do so. It might feel too comfortable. On the other hand, if they are too difficult, you will not be successful and become frustrated by failing and eventually give up! You don't want to fall into either trap. Let me give you some examples of good SMART goals and ones that just don't cut it.

Good specific goal: I will take a 15-minute walk during my lunch break on Monday, Wednesday, and Friday.

Poorly written goal: I will walk more this week.

Good specific goal: I will make a fruit and veggie shake for my breakfast at least three days this week and take it with me on my ride to work.

Poorly written goal: I am going to drink more healthy shakes this week.

Good specific goal: I will work on losing 2 pounds this week by increasing my activity to 4 days a week and by counting my calories using MyFitnessPal every day.

Poorly written goal: I will lose 2 pounds this week.

Get the idea? You need to be as specific as possible indicating how often, when, and how much.

If you find yourself being vague, ask yourself what "more" or "less" means. It is not good enough to say that you will exercise "more" or smoke "less"; be specific! Once you do this, you will need to make sure it is realistic and that you are fairly confident that you have a shot at success. You do this by gauging your comfort level on a scale of 1-10 with 1 being not confident at all and 10 being extremely confident. If you are a 5 or below, you need to reevaluate your goal and make changes so that you feel more confident. Ultimately, you should be a 6-10 to have the most successful outcomes with your goals. Many of my clients started at a 4 or a 5 when making their first set of Weekly Goals. When this happened I asked them, "So, what do we need to change to make that number higher?" They would then think about it and come up with an answer fairly quickly, such as changing the amount of time exercising or the amount of days doing something. Think about this on your own when you are constructing your Weekly Goals and be sure that you are asking yourself to stretch slightly outside your comfort zone, but not so much that it feels almost impossible. Remember, the key to goal setting, and the reason why we do it, is to have success so that it improves your self-efficacy and gives you the momentum to move forward towards your Wellness Vision! Setting lofty goals that are never attained will only set you up for failure; so let's get off to the right start here and now. Stop here and begin setting 1-3 Weekly Goals for yourself. Practice writing and rewriting them until they sound specific enough and you feel confident that you will be able to give it your best shot. Stop here and come back when you are ready……

- Okay, *really*, stop here and take some time to think about and develop your baby steps towards your future wellness! Don't rush this task; take a few minutes or a few hours to really dig deep and think about what you want to accomplish this week. Does it seem doable or are you trying to do too much too soon?

(You will also have more time to practice goal setting in the case study.)

Now that you have had some time to practice your first attempts at weekly goal writing, and you have already worked on your Wellness Vision and 3-Month Goals, let's talk a little bit about keeping everything in perspective. After all, this is the real world. Since most people are concerned about fitness and dietary habits, let's think about what is realistic in these areas. Before you go off the deep end and tell yourself that you are going to clean out the pantry of all "bad" foods and that you will resign yourself to exercise 7 days a week, let's put the brakes on and do a reality check. Ask yourself; are your expectations realistic? Is only eating "clean" foods 100% of the time what we do in the real world? Is working out 7 days a week without any rest really good for your body? The answer to all of these questions is "no". This is life, and in this life we crave certain foods and folks generally either don't work out at all, or try to do too much too soon. So, before we go any further, here are a few words about nutrition and too much exercise, since many of you will be constructing your goals around these areas.

Some of us crave sweets that are gooey goodness, and others crave salty snack foods or fried delicacies, or anything made out of bacon. Is this wrong? Are we doomed to a life of never eating what we love? Of course not! In the real world we indulge, but we just learn how to do it better and with more self- control so that we can still enjoy food but not sabotage our wellness efforts. For starters just try to take time to be more mindful about good food choices and practice portion control. (More tips coming in later chapters.)

With regard to exercise, many people have the all or nothing attitude. "If 4 days is good then 7 is the best!" Many of my clients also think if high intensity training is good for two days a week then 5 is even better! Not so!

Your body needs a break, even when you are trying to lose a few pounds. You cannot work it every day and expect to glean fabulous results. You need to rest, and rest is just as important as your workouts. For instance, your "off" days from weight training are when your muscles rebuild and repair in order to become bigger muscles, and the time you take to rest from cardio workouts is when your system gets a break from all of the hard work you have been putting it through, which lessons the likelihood for injury and constant soreness.

Start by doing 2 or 3 days of exercise a week and then build up. Just keep it simple! And, no need to do HIIT all the time!

- Quick point: The whole idea of High Intensity Interval Training (HIIT) is to shock the system and force your body to work at its highest level, but only for short bursts of time in a <u>shorter</u> workout. Doing this 2-3 times a week can increase fat and calorie burn, but doing it more than that can cause your body to become used to it negating its effects, or even worse, you can injure yourself!

So, go all the way back to your Wellness Vision and make sure to do a reality check with all of your hopes and dreams of the future before moving on.

This is a very important first step that you need to spend some time on before getting too far into the change process. If you have unrealistic expectations or have put too many goals into play, you need to reel it in.

It's important to not put so much pressure on yourself; no one is perfect, no one eats perfectly all the time (if they do they are not fun to hang out with), and no one works out constantly without some ill effects. We are the average "Joe" with normal lives; we we need to figure out how to make wellness fit our own livestyle in a realistic, gradual, uncomplicated way. Change is taking you out of your comfort zone; so by making it as uncomplicated and comfortable as possible, the more likely these changes will become newer, better, lifetime habits!

A good vision, with stable real-world goals to get you there, are the steps needed to do this once and for all. You <u>will</u> make changes, one step at a time. This time, you will do it!

So, I think it might be a good idea to take a look at a mock client. Well, not really a mock client, but a scenario culminating from many clients that I have had over the years; a scenario that covers a lot of surface area and will speak to many of you reading this book. We will review the case of Mary. Mary is a 48-year-old woman who works as an office assistant in a local doctor's office. She has fairly stable hours and is able to take a full 30-minute lunch break every day. She told me that her job is very hectic and quite often she gets stressed over the patients who call with complaints or who have to reschedule at the last minute. Overall though, she said she does like what she does and enjoys her coworkers; some of whom have become close friends over the years. She has been married to her husband for 20 years and they have two children ages 15 and 12. The family is often very busy due to sports, so they are traveling from game to game during the week, often eating out or grabbing something at a convenience store. Mary told me that they only eat at home 2-3 nights a week, and many times they do not have time to fully plan a dinner so it might be just frozen lasagna. She stated that she used to go to the workout room at the hospital during her lunch break or after her shift, but has since stopped doing it and is not sure why. After work is normally not an option due to the hectic family schedule, but she stated that she could possibly use her lunch break to get some exercise. Mary said her main goal is to lose weight and learn what to eat, but she is afraid that she will have to learn how to do all of these things, which seems like a lot, and simply won't be able to find the time.

I asked Mary if there was ever a time in her life when she did feel healthy and her weight was where she wanted it to be. She said that it had been during her 20s when she and her husband were dating. She weighed about 130 pounds and the two of them hiked a lot and went on canoe trips. They had only the two of them to worry about, so their schedule was less hectic and they ate at home almost every night. She said those were some of the best times in her life and she felt fit and in control. When I asked her what changes she would like to see in the next 6-12 months, she stated that she just wants to put herself first a little more often. She would like to be able to be more organized and begin to eat healthier, even though life gets busy. Within a year she would like to have several healthy "go to" dinners that she and her family can enjoy. Since she feels that she has a lack of time, she wants to work on finding ways to organize her time more efficiently and set a schedule for herself that includes weekly workouts.

After speaking with Mary at her first appointment and hearing about her lifestyle, two words seemed to sum up everything: busy and unorganized. Would you agree? I bet a lot of you are in the same position as Mary. It seems that everything else comes before you and your needs. When you *do* decide to make somewhat of a plan, the first person who needs that block of time with you will automatically get it, and everything else gets thrown out the window. Although you would like to eat better and make healthier choices, there are always pitfalls that lie in wait such as the office break room or the neighbor's BBQ weekends. Your time and energy always seems to be focused on something outside of yourself. Well let me tell you, it is time to put yourself first! Right here and now! You can actually make lifetime changes; it just takes a bit of effort and some well-planned baby steps each week. Mary did it, and so can you!

After reviewing the key points in my notes, the first thing I asked Mary to do was to think about what was most important to her and to come up with some positive action statements to begin forming her Wellness Vision. She came up with several things that she felt were attainable by the one year mark, and things that she knew she wanted to take time to work on. Here is her Wellness Vision:

"I am a fit and active person who is 18 pounds lighter and has a new way of seeing the world. I am happy and my family is happy. We do outdoor activities on the weekends such as canoeing and hiking, as well as play sports as a family to help the kids practice. After telling my family that I needed help getting organized, all three have been chipping in to make sure healthy snacks are prepared each day and equipment is ready to go when we have our outings, or when we go to practice during the week. I am also committed to working out during my lunch break and have even gotten some of my office friends on board. Doing this has helped with my stress levels and allows me to cope much better with the difficult patients. I never realized how much exercise can help relieve stress! When I do face challenges, my motivation to feel the zest for life as I did in my 20s keeps me going, and my

family continues to be supportive and involved in the
process. Eating healthy, exercising, and having a
more organized household are important to me and is
within my grasp. Doing all of these things has helped
keep the stress levels at bay and also makes me feel
like I am meeting all of my needs, finally!
Life is good!"

Wow, what a great start! This Wellness Vision gives Mary a clear path towards her positive future. Initially, the key here will be to read and re-read this statement to begin to plant the seed in her mind so that it can begin to sprout. You will be surprised how this simple first step will begin to transform your decision-making during the first few days. And as you already learned, you will begin to start breaking down this idea into more manageable steps by taking pieces from your Wellness Vision and creating a

3-Month Goal. I asked Mary to do this; I asked her what she felt she could realistically accomplish by the three- month mark and to come up with several statements indicating exactly what she will be doing by that point in time. Here is what she came up with: 3-Month Goal:

I am walking for 20 minutes during my lunch break 3 to 4 days a week, and have even gotten some of my coworkers on board. Three days a week I substitute my workplace lunch with a salad I bring from home. I also bring two healthy snacks on those same days. I am down 10 pounds since month 2 and have continued to stay on track by losing 1-2 pounds per week. I have done this by doing my lunchtime workouts as well as the changes I made in my diet.

This is a wonderful shorter-term goal for Mary and I was impressed with how she took segments of her Wellness Vision and broke down some of the goals into smaller pieces that she felt she could accomplish within three months.

You will do the same with your 3-Month Goal; look at your Wellness Vision again and take 3 or 4 key points from it to devise some smaller steps you can take. Where will you be at the 3-month mark? What will you be doing by that time? Use Mary's example to help you; perhaps you will simply rewrite some of the ideas you already wrote down. Remember, always keep it positive and keep it in the present tense. These statements are the foundation for the final step that we take on the road to change; the Weekly Goals, which you can think of as your baby steps. Let's begin the weekly goal process with Mary!

You will now begin to take specific actions in order to start reaching the 3-Month Goals you have set for yourself, which are ultimately part of the big picture; the Wellness Vision!

Taking parts of your 3-Month Goals and breaking them down further enables you to start the process of change. Let's discuss how to formulate the Weekly Goals appropriately. We will be using the S.M.A.R.T. method. These are your baby steps on the road to success and the final part of the goal-setting process!

SMART stands for:

S: Specific

M: Measurable

A: Action-Based

R: Realistic

T: Time-Lined

We use this type of goal setting to further break down your larger goals you have set for the 3-month point. You should include only one measurable behavior per goal and make sure you feel fairly confident that you can reach it. The goal needs to be as specific as possible and give the *how* and *when* aspects such as "3 times a week" or "on my lunch break". Again, you should stretch *just beyond* what you are comfortable doing so that you can improve your success rate and self-efficacy. (This is the feeling of confidence and belief in yourself that you glean from achieving your goals, and helps perpetuate a higher self-esteem.)

I hope I haven't lost you yet; I know it might sound a little confusing at first. But don't worry, I am going to give you some examples of the types of Weekly Goals Mary used to get herself started on her wellness journey so you will have a clear idea of what is expected. Here we go…

Weekly Goal 1: I will walk around the parameter of the campus during my lunch break for 15 minutes three days a week with my coworker Kim.

Weekly Goal 2: I will take 2 healthy snacks to work 2 days this week. I will choose from yogurt, veggies and dip, and almonds.

Weekly Goal 3: I will plan 3 easy-prep dinners on Sunday evening so I know what to cook when I get home from work during the week. I will go to the store on Monday after work to pick up everything that I need for the week.

Now go back and notice how these goals correlate to her 3-Month Goal, as well as the *big picture* Wellness Vision. She is breaking it down and taking small steps towards the larger goals of the future. This is what you need to do to be successful with your behavior change process. The key is to take it step by step and clearly define your goals for each of the processes that we have discussed. Some coaching manuals recommend between 2-5 goals each week, I however, have had the most success by limiting my clients to 3 goals.

I found that if a person had more than that, there was a greater chance of failure with one or more of the goals. It is better to stick with 1-3 and feel fairly confident that you will at least try to complete them rather than putting too much on your plate. (No pun intended!)

At no time should you feel overburdened by your goals. Use the scale of 1-10 when thinking about your confidence level for completing the goal. One (1) is not confident at all, and 10 is extremely confident. Your Weekly Goals should be no lower than a 6. Otherwise, revamp your goal so you feel more confident about it. Not having confidence in your goals will only set you up for failure in your attempts and continue to keep you from attaining successful change. Be sure to use your scale of 1-10 with each of your Weekly Goals and be honest with yourself.

Let me give you an example: At first, Mary wanted to go "all in" with her lunchtime walking goal and thought it might be best to jump in with both feet first! Initially, this is what she said. "My goal is to walk the parameter of the building for 20 minutes 3 times a week during lunch with my coworker Kim."

But when I asked what her confidence number was, she said "4". After talking with her about it, she said that she really did not know if she could do all three days because this was a busy week at work with some yearly reports that needed to be completed and meetings that she needed to attend; some meetings might cut into her lunch hour. I asked her what it would take to make her goal feel more "doable" and she came up with a better version of it. "I will walk around the parameter of the campus during my lunch break for 15 minutes two days a week with my coworker Kim." Mary then felt she was a "7" with her confidence because she knew that if a meeting ran over, she would still be able to fit in 15 minutes of walking, as well as have time to eat something afterward. She also felt that she could more easily commit to do it at least 2 days instead of 3.

Now it is time for you to put this into action! You should have already written your Wellness Vison paragraph and then broken that down to your smaller 3-Month Goal. Now, what did you decide to do *this* week to start taking baby steps? What is it that you can do right now to begin the change process? If you haven't already, write down at least 2 things that you want to try for your goals this week. Write your sentences using the S.M.A.R.T methodology and make sure your confidence number is at least a "6". You now have completed all three steps in the goal-setting process! The Weekly Goals are the starting point for your steps towards lifetime changes! So, go ahead and get started on your path towards change! You can do this!

Chapter 5

Falling off the wagon:

Strategies for continued success

Okay, so now that you have a solid foundation with a Wellness Vision and goal setting strategies, let's talk about staying on track and making things stick. There are several tools to keep you motivated in the maintenance stage, as well as behavior strategies to help you continue to get what you want and need, and to keep you motivated. Let's start with two big ones; *saying no* and *asking for what you need.* It's time to face the fact that you cannot be everything to everyone all of the time. It is impossible! Trying to do this creates a vacuum of stress and failed attempts at providing for your own needs. Your energy is being sucked right out of you and you have nothing left for yourself! Well, that is about to change. Let's first talk about learning to say "no" and then "asking for what you need. By using these two tools, you will set yourself up for success and be able to thrive!

Saying "no" is the starting point for this process because it sets limits and allows you to take control of your decision making. When was the last time you said "no" to a friend or family member?

When you were asked to pick up your friend's kids after school even though you had errands of your own to do, what was your answer? When your boss asked if you could work the weekend shift for the rest of the month, which was the only time with your kids, how did you respond? Too many people simply agree to all requests and take on tasks and responsibilities that they really don't have time for or *want* to do. The same can be said for food choices. Remember that dinner party you went to that had all those delectable deserts? You limited yourself to one and had your favorite brownie; then, your best friend asked you to try a slice of her blueberry pie. What did you say?

Saying "no" is not being rude, it is telling the truth and not allowing yourself to take on too much or give into temptations. Let me give you some ideas about how you can say "no" in these situations.

"Sorry, I have a lot of errands to do today, but I could help you out later this week." "No, I cannot work every weekend this month; it is the only time I have with my kids. I can work a few extra hours during the week if that helps." "No thank you, I allowed myself one dessert for this party and I have already had it."

Now YOU try it! The only way your life will be less stressful and chaotic is if you change the way you do things. Saying "no" is one of the first steps in the process.

- Stop here and ponder this idea for a few minutes, or a few days. Write down the first situations that come to mind where you have trouble saying "no", and then create sentences that will work for you in those situations.

Now, what about your needs; are they being met? Why not? Well, perhaps those around you don't know what you want because you have never told them! Maybe they do not understand how to support you while you strive to become healthier and more fit. They are not mind readers; they don't always know what you want! It's time to change that. You will start to get what you want and need when you *ask for it*!

Here are the three key starter phrases:
I feel...

I need…
Would you please…

Again, you are not being rude. It is not rude to state your thoughts, feelings, needs, and problems. Here are examples of how this might work for you.

I feel very unhealthy with the food choices I have been making, and feel tempted when it is right in front of me.

I need both of us to keep junk out of the house.

Would you please keep cookies and candy at your office instead of here at the house, or not buy it in the first place?

You are stating YOUR feelings and YOUR needs using "I" statements, which is what makes it work! Now, try this on your own. Say "no" to situations and choices that are not good for you. Tell the people around you what you need and how you feel so that they can help you on your wellness journey.
It is all about communication.

Take some time to think of examples of how you can say "no" to various requests. Then fill out your "I feel" "I need" and "Would you please" statements to help you get what you are looking for. You will find that when you learn to take on less of what other people are asking of you and be true to yourself, you will be a much happier and less stressed person.

- Stop here and write down your own sentences using the provided phrases to help you feel more confident about telling people what you need. It is important to practice these skills to become more adept at using them when the time comes.

Now, what happens when you have a bad day, a bad week, or a fleeting moment of self-doubt; how can you keep that positive dialog going on in your head? We all have that nagging negative voice that tells us we "don't belong" or we are "never going to lose this weight"; it is a normal part of the human psyche. But this does not mean we have to let it run rampant!

Cognitive reframing, or reconstruction, is a way to help you change your negative self-talk into more positive experiences. Cognitive reframing is a psychological technique that identifies and then disputes the negative thought running through your mind. It is a way to view the experience or thought in a more positive way.

To put it simply, you are *changing* the way you look at something! Doing this allows you to challenge the negative thought and become a more positive and happy person; no more negative voice! Okay, if it were that easy none of us would ever fall victim to the negative junk we say to ourselves. The real point of this exercise is to begin to be more aware of your negative voice and then to practice reframing the voice into something more positive.

This will take time; some negative thoughts or past hurts run very deep. You will find that sometimes it is easy and other times you really need to work at it until it finally sticks. Simply repeating the new, positive phrase to yourself is what will make it part of your new habit. Okay, so let's talk about what we need to do first.

Step 1: As soon as the negative thought pops into your head, stop; does your perception match the reality? Is what you are thinking or saying to yourself really true? Probably not. "I didn't lose two pounds this week so this is never going to work." "NEVER GOING TO WORK." How realistic is that? Not very.

Step 2: Once you stop yourself dead in your thought–processing tracks and identify that you have a negative message coming through, the next step is to try to see it in a more positive light.

What did you learn from the experience? When did you have success in the past? Draw from these questions to reframe your self-talk.

"This was a rough week but I learned that I need to be more organized so I have healthy options on hand when it is time to make dinner and prepare snacks. Next week I will do better!"

The bottom line is that being aware and more mindful of our negative thoughts is the first step in stopping them; then restructuring and deciding what thoughts you are going to let in will be the next step to help squelch the negative voice that is running rampant. Remember, seeing something as positive or negative is a choice; it is up to you to make the right choice! Take some time to think about what you say to yourself each day, and become more aware when those thoughts need to be changed.

- Stop here and try this: Think of 2-3 negative thoughts that your negative voice keeps feeding you. Work on reframing these thoughts into something better that you can let in and become part of your positive self-talk.

Keep these positive sentences in the forefront of your mind by writing them down and posting them in your high-traffic areas; office desk, bathroom mirror, refrigerator, or car. The more positive thoughts you read and re-read to yourself every day, the sooner *they* will be running rampant through your mind rather than the negative junk. That was your old story; now you are embarking on a new and positive journey. Have fun with the reframing process and keep practicing!

Falling off the proverbial wagon is something else that happens to everyone. Sometimes we find ourselves doing the same things over and over again and losing sight of our long-range plan. We all need to keep our vision in sight and stay connected to our plan. Staying connected to your overall master plan can help you avoid this pitfall. If you see yourself achieving success and keeping your eye on the prize, it will be much easier to stay on the wagon and continue on your journey. *If you see it you can be it!* Let's talk more about this simple phrase that sets the tone for success! So far we talked a lot about goal setting in this book, and as you have read in the beginning, you learned why the process of creating a Wellness Vision is so important. Seeing yourself in the future is a monumental component of helping you stick to and achieve your goals in the here and now.

As mentioned, your vision should be specific and clear and embody what you want to have achieved by a certain point in time, usually 1 year is a good place to start. You also set 3-Month Goals and Weekly Goals that are both stepping stones leading up to our Wellness Vision. Goal setting is an important part of your vision; it is *how* you achieve something. The vision is the big picture; think of the vision as the *why*.

Let's focus on this. What do you want out of life? Where do you want to be? What do you want to look and feel like? Why? These are all questions that need to be answered when developing your long-term plan of where you are and *why*. Now think about this and read your vision, picture yourself in that place doing the things you are saying, and looking like the best version of yourself.

It is so important to actually *see* yourself doing the things that are in your vision; the mind is a very powerful tool and can help lead you towards your goals. Close your eyes and see yourself a different shape than you are now. *Feel* the energy of your newly-found activity level. *Smell* and taste the healthier foods that you are putting on the table and into your body.

The point is to *really* think that this is already happening and you are there in that very moment. Now you have planted the seed in your mind that will begin to grow! *Seeing* it is your first step! Now let's take this a step further. It might be difficult for you to always find that place in your mind to envision your positive future self, especially if you haven't read your vision in a while, so let's make a visual that is always right in front of you.

Creating a **vision board** is a perfect way to keep in mind what you are setting out to do every day! Use a piece of cardboard or construction paper to adhere words, pictures, slogans, and sayings that exemplify what you want for your future. It can be anything; just make sure it speaks to what your vision is all about. This vision board can be simple and take just a few minutes leafing through a magazine for pictures, or you can take an entire week to put it together using various items that showcase your dreams. Be creative and make sure to put it in a place where you can see it every day as a reminder of where you WILL be in the future.

Seeing your vision every day will help that seed to grow and before you know it, the future you will be in full bloom!

Another wonderful tool to use later in your journey is self-mentoring. Mentoring others who are in the initial stages of change just as you once were is a great motivational tool! When you start to consider yourself an old hat and a near-pro with reaching wellness goals, it is a great time for you to teach and lead others by example, as well as talking about what you have learned. Now, this is not to say that you should go around spewing forth a know-it-all attitude with those who are still greenhorns, but rather, being there as a supporter for a friend or coworker as they begin their journey. You now have many of the tools that they might be looking for!

Ask them if they would like some seasoned advice or just someone to work out with and be accountable to. They will probably be excited to have a workout partner and happy that you are taking interest in them.

Teaching someone else or just being their workout buddy is a huge motivator to keep you on track for the long haul. Keep this in mind as you come across friends and family who are embarking on the same journey you were on. It will make you feel great that you can help them out, and also keep yourself on the straight and narrow at the same time!

Lastly, some people are motivated by larger goals. You might be the type who always needs an event or new "big thing" planned for the future to keep your eye on. Many of my clients turn into race junkies, as they are always planning their next big event! Scheduling fitness goals such as a 5K or bike-a-thon is a super way for those who are motivated by events to keep a steady course through the maintenance stage. Many of my clients have become avid triathletes and look forward to each upcoming race and the training that precedes it. Some of my clients join Masters teams for swimming or running. Whatever event strikes your fancy, just get out there and do it.

Staying motivated is all about knowing what tactics best suit you and trying new ones to keep the process fresh! New workouts, different venues, fresh recipes, new visions, and major athletic events can be implemented in the maintenance stage to keep you moving forward. Let's keep the new you rocking!

Chapter 6

Tips, tools, and more tweaks:

Adding to your lifetime toolbox

When I finish with a coaching client the normal end-of-session question is, "Is there anything else I should know?" By this time, my clients have the tools they need to succeed, but what they need to know is how to remind themselves of what to do when the going gets tough; which tool to take out and when! No matter what tools you are using, the whole works can get gummed up by one thing: your negative voice. Your negative self-talk is probably the biggest bully that you will deal with both during and after your transformation. (Even when you have attained many of your goals and are in the maintenance stage, your negative voice can still try to derail you!) The most important thing to remember is to continuously feed yourself with positivity! Every time that negativity rears its ugly head, you need to have a rebuttal ready to go. (Revisit the idea about reframing that I mentioned earlier.) Let's review this a moment: Here is what you might say to yourself when things are not going well. "You didn't lose any weight this week; this is never going to work." That is simply not true! So you had an off week, so what!? Rephrase this to reflect a more positive mind set. "I maintained my weight this week and I can feel my body changing. I will continue to make better choices and I know this weight will come off!" It takes some effort, and you need to allow time for this new habit to stick just like any other, but keep trying and review the reframing steps mentioned in chapter 5. Stay positive!

If you are having trouble coming up with your own positive, motivating statements, here is a list of some you can use or tweak to fit your needs. Just make sure you are reading these words or statements to yourself every day. Place them somewhere where you will see them such as on the refrigerator, on the bathroom mirror, or in your cubicle at work! Plant that positive seed in your mind! Let's go!

Positive Statements

If you see it you can be it!

Change your thoughts, change your life!
–Dr. Wayne Dyer

I am capable of achieving anything!

A journey of a thousand miles begins with a single step. – Confucius

I know I am stronger than I think I am!

You can do this!

Faith is taking the first step even when you don't see the whole staircase.–Martin Luther King Jr.

I am bigger than this temptation; I will prevail!

Today is a brand new day!

I feel energized and ready for the challenge!

Yes I can!

This is only a small sample of the positive statements that you might use for your daily self-talk. Search the internet, look in books or poems, and find a few that resonate with you then continue to repeat them to yourself when that negativity tries to get in your way. Staying on track and making your habits stick depends on *you* and the process you learned about in this book. Remember your three main tools for success: your Wellness Vision, the 3-Month Goal, and your Weekly Goals. From time to time you will need to re-evaluate your vision and goals, especially when you start to achieve what you have initially set out to do.

If you have been working on specific goals for over 3 months, make sure you are checking in with yourself and seeing whether or not you have achieved what you set out to do by that point, or if you need to make changes with a new 3-Month Plan.

Changes might need to be made and a new 3-Month Goal with associated Weekly Goals will need to be established. During this time, you might suddenly realize that you have been on track and doing this for several months! Congratulations; you are in the maintenance stage! Let's talk more about this important stage of change and discuss additional strategies that will keep you on track.

One of the last conversations my clients and I have involves discussing how to keep things fresh so they can continue in the maintenance stage and maintain their new lifestyle habits. Here are some reminders that will help you maintain your results. Remember, you always need to keep your eye on the prize! It can be easy to get off track when you no longer see or think about your vision for the future, so it is important to have those visual reminders in high-traffic areas of your home. Type or write your vision and put it at your desk at work, have a copy on the fridge, or set it as a reminder in your phone that pops up every day!

Now that you are in the maintenance stage of your behavior, you also need to think about what will continue to drive you forward so that you keep the momentum going for the long run. As I already mentioned, revamping your Wellness Vision and creating new goals will help to keep you excited about moving forward; it is important to have motivators to keep you interested. Perhaps now is the time to sign up for that 5K you have always thought about, or take the yoga class that your friends always wanted you to join. Reach a little further than you think is possible. At this point, you have more self-efficacy and feel like you can accomplish what you set out to do, so stretching beyond the norm may be a little easier in this stage. You now have formed some solid habits and it is time to reach outside of yourself for continued motivation.

Another tool that was briefly mentioned earlier is thinking about YOU becoming the teacher! Yes, you! You may not think you are capable of taking on this role but don't sell yourself short; you now have what it takes to help gently push others in the right direction. Start a walking group, talk with a friend about how to set realistic goals, show someone how to revamp a recipe to make it healthier; whatever you do, just pass on your knowledge and enthusiasm and be their supporter. This not only helps others get onto the wellness bandwagon, but it is also a strong motivational tool for you as well!

Be advised that plateauing is prevalent at this juncture. When maintaining your new habits, be careful that your exercise routine or diet does not become stagnant. Simply being a mentor might very well help to prevent you from getting bored with what you have been doing, but for most of my wellness clients, exercise is the first thing that becomes hum drum and uninteresting. Remember to keep your workouts fresh! The reason why people hit a plateau is because they do the same exercise all of the time with little or no variation. It is imperative to keep a check on your routine and up the ante every couple of months so that your body continues to adapt.

Let's get into some specifics about what you can change.

Perhaps you are ready to increase the amount of weight you are using, do more repetitions, or more sets. Maybe you need to add a few different cardiovascular workouts like a step class or HIIT mix to your schedule. Many times when we reach this stagnancy of a plateau, it has a lot to do with how we are moving our bodies (or not) and what types of exercise we are engaging in. If you have been doing the same routine for 6 months or more, without changing any aspect of it, you are more than likely not seeing any major results. For instance, steady-state cardio is great, but if this is all you are doing you might want to spice things up a bit. If results are what you are looking for, look no further than High Intensity Interval Training or HIIT.

This type of workout helps you burn additional calories and supercharges your metabolism and overall endurance in a shorter workout session. In this workout, you are interchanging between a mild to moderate movement and a burst of higher intensity that lasts anywhere from 15-30 seconds (or more) with a total workout time of 20-30 minutes.

How many bursts you do and how intense they are depends on your fitness level and experience. There is a lot of flexibility with HIIT, as you can utilize its strategy with anything you are doing: walking on the treadmill, running outdoors, riding a stationary bike, or using a step bench. Simply add a couple of bursts to your workout and see how you do; you can then add more as time goes on. Interval workouts can be added a few times a week to spice up your exercise routine; however, take it slow and always get a doctor's approval if you are new to exercise or if you have any medical issues.

What else needs to change when you are in the maintenance stage? Perhaps it is time to change your menu and try some new recipes! What we eat and how much of it definitely affects our fitness goals and ultimately how much we weigh. In the past three decades, there has been an increase in processed foods, fast food restaurants, and super-sizing of portions. Besides being nutritionally deficient, many of today's food choices dish up much larger portions than they used to and our waistlines have been paying the price!

By making a few simple changes to your dietary routine, you can keep these calories in check, watch your portions, and put more nutrient-rich foods into your diet.

Sometimes all it takes is knowing exactly *what* you are putting into your body. One thing that works wonders for most everyone is food journaling.

By keeping track of your daily food intake, portions, and calories, you are less likely to overeat. It is amazing how this simple task can be so effective in reducing daily calories and preventing you from eating so much junk; you simply don't want to write it down! (Try the My Fitness Pal app or the trackers on Choosemyplate.gov to keep track of your foods. Both of these sites are listed in Chapter 8.)

Also, adding more veggies to your day lowers your overall calorie intake and gives you a burst of nutrients that your body craves. Try to keep cut up carrots, cukes, broccoli, and bell peppers handy in your fridge so that you can dip them in hummus or low-fat dressing for your snacks, or use them in salads. Use fruits and veggies in your smoothies for an easy and delicious way to get more nutrients into your day. However you can get more fruits and veggies into your day, do it!

Another thing to remember is portion control, especially if you are eating outside the home. If you are out for dinner, watch those portions! As mentioned earlier, portion sizes have increased tremendously over the decades; we simply do not need THAT much food! Try sharing your meal, get an appetizer instead of a main dish, or ask for a *to-go* container as soon as they bring your entree and place half of your meal in it to take home. If you try any of the nutritional strategies listed, you will surely be on your way to making lasting changes and you will see and feel a difference in your body.

Still, there are many reasons why people become stagnant in their fitness regimen and stand happily (or not so much) on the plateau just plugging along; our behavior, our exercise routine, and our nutritional habits are a few of the biggest players. But if you take a serious look at these areas and try to make one or two changes at a time, you will most certainly find yourself stepping beyond the plateau.

Remember, it's not about doing everything all at once; don't bite off more than you can chew, literally! Take small steps towards changing your behavior by choosing 1 or 2 areas to work on. Whatever area of wellness, just make sure you tweak your Vision and Goals from time to time so you are less likely to get stuck in the stagnant waters of boredom and hit a plateau.

The key to your success is to first <u>know what you want</u> and to make sure it is <u>you</u> making the decision. When you have this as your first step, you will be heading in the right direction for the right reasons. Setting realistic goals is key to ensuring your success, and staying on track involves using the tools discussed to keep things fresh and exciting as you continue on your journey. Now is the time for change, now is your time to shine! This time you are going to make wellness work!

Chapter 7

Top 5 Tips for Getting Back on Track

Plus, Surviving the Holidays

Think of this chapter as your fast track to getting BACK on track! Whenever you feel that you have had a slight slip in your plan, jump start your journey once again by following these "doable" tips. Let's keep it plain and simple; here are **five** things you can do today to help shed weight and start to get back on track with your behavior goals. Soon you will be feeling fit and fabulous in no time!

1. Drink lemon water every day. Start your day with a glass of lemon water by squeezing a couple of wedges into a glass and filling it with ice cold water. Not only is it refreshing and hydrating for your body, it aides digestion and cleanses the system. Lemon water also helps to fight bloat during the day, as it is a natural diuretic and also helps to curb your appetite.

The toxin-fighting lemon also packs a wallop of vitamin C, which is especially helpful in the cold and flu season. In short, lemons are amazing. What more do I need to say? Start drinking lemon water today!

2. Increase you veggie intake. Nothing packs the nutritional punch like veggies! Try to get as many into your day as possible by adding them into every meal and for your snacks. Don't like vegetables? No problem! You can hide them in your morning smoothie. If you have never tried it, this is a fantastic way to add vitamin-rich foods to your day without even tasting them! Simply throw a little kale and/or baby spinach into the blender along with your fruits and protein powder; you will never know they are there. If you do have a palette for veggies, replace some of your non-

nutritive snacks with carrot sticks, pepper slices, or cauliflower with low fat dip or hummus. The more veggies you put into your day the more satisfied you will feel, and you will begin to see the pounds drop off in no time!

3. Change the intensity of your workout. As mentioned previously, if you have been doing the same type of cardiovascular exercise for several months without changing any aspect of it, you are more than likely not seeing any major results. Steady-state exercise is great, but if this is all you are doing you might want to spice things up a bit. High Intensity Interval Training or HIIT is an awesome addition to any workout routine to do just that! This type of workout allows you to increase

your metabolism both during and after your workout for up to 12 hours afterwards! High intensity workouts are where you are putting forth the most effort possible for a short period of time. You are interchange between these high intensity bursts and rest periods and do this for only 30 minutes or less. The more intense your workout bursts, the shorter the workout should be. Because this is a more aggressive (although shorter workout) this should only be done 1-3 times a week to prevent injury, or for the workouts to lose their effectiveness. Try a HIIT workout this week and begin to change up your routine!

4.   Eat your largest meal in the middle of the day. The Europeans do it, and overall, they are much slimmer and healthier than most

Americans. Eating your largest meal in the middle of the day just makes sense; you are most active during the day and therefore have plenty of time to burn off those excess calories. You will also feel more satisfied and most likely will not have that mid-afternoon crash at the office anymore. By the time you are ready for dinner, a smaller, simpler meal will usually suffice; think salad, yogurt and berries, or one of those smoothies I mentioned in tip number two. This can shave off tremendous amounts of excess calories, especially when you think about the 7-8 hours of fasting your body goes through every night after your last meal. Try this a few days a week and you will soon wake up seeing and feeling a difference!

5. Be more mindful. Being mindful is simply being more aware of what is happening in the present moment; taking a step back, taking a deep breath, and taking in the here and now. Being mindful is all about being aware of what you are thinking, feeling, and doing right now and possibly asking yourself "why". This not only helps you to slow down a little during the day, but also helps when you are trying to understand yourself in the midst of behavior change. Being mindful can help us to make better choices, as it helps us to slow down our thoughts and check in with our true feelings. If we really think about our level of hunger and why we are reaching for a certain type of food, we might make a different choice. People often use this technique when they are

trying to break a bad habit; being more mindful of why they smoke a cigarette, what makes them stressed, or why they avoid exercise, can shed some light on why we have certain behaviors, and in turn, it helps us to change them and start adopting new ways of *being*. It all begins with mindfulness.

So, there are your top 5 game changers, but now here it is, the biggest road-block and the one thing that can derail people faster than a speeding locomotive: The Holidays! We all know the holidays come up fast and there are sure to be just as many temptations, excuses, and overindulgences we expect as every year. So, what's your plan *this* time? How will you do it differently? Might I suggest *being prepared*?

During my many years as a Girl Scout from ages 7-16, I think I heard this mantra at least 600 times! It was the foundation for what we Scouts stood for; being organized and ready for the unexpected! This mantra has carried over into my adult life, and although I have been "Type A" all of my life, I think that I would still "be prepared" even if I was more laid back due to it being drilled into my head for so many years. It is my belief that the more prepared you are the better the outcome. Period.

Being prepared, especially around the holidays is of the utmost importance for anyone who has a pulse; but especially for those who are working on health and wellness issues such as diet, exercise, and stress reduction. What is your plan for this holiday season?

How will you handle those blips in your schedule that throw everything off kilter? What will you do with all of the sweet treats and rich desserts that everyone keeps dropping off at your office in festive little tins? Now is the time to create your plan of action! Nothing is going to throw you off track *this* time; <u>nothing</u>! And, I am here to help you create a plan to Be Prepared! Here are some tips:

First: Think about what you do and don't have control over. Create a schedule that is loosely based upon the things that you can control, but leave a little wiggle room for the unexpected dramas that might pop up. For example, schedule some "you" time in the morning and get your workout finished so that when schedule changes come up later in the day you will not make an excuse as to why you didn't have time to exercise. (Sound familiar?)

Second: Refer back to my message about saying "no". This will be one of the best times of year to start using your voice to state what you want and need, as well as saying "no" to things that create stress around the holidays. Just Say No!

Third: Select a few staple holiday recipes that you and your family enjoy each season, and give them a re-do! There is always a way to reduce the fat and calories in our favorite foods, and revamping old family favorites is a great way to keep them on the menu, but feel better about partaking of them. Using skim milk instead of whole, apple sauce instead of oil, reduced fat cheese instead of regular, are just a few simple tweaks to get you started. Try Googling the recipe and type "low calorie" or "low fat" in your search and you will come up with tons of options!

Now, it is your turn! I want to you begin to prepare for your holiday journey by thinking about any potential barriers to your success and prepare for them. Write down your concerns and come up with solutions so you're prepared and ready for battle!

- Okay, time to stop again! Take a moment to work up a simple plan or schedule that you will use for the holidays. What specifically will you do differently? How will you be more prepared?

Chapter 8

Final Thoughts and Fitness Resources

At some point in the process, you may wish to work with a personal trainer, wellness coach, or other health professional in order to stay on track. Working one-on-one with a professional will help keep you accountable, and in some cases is the one thing that can keep people on track and moving forward. Be careful about who you choose to guide you. The person should be professional and certified in the appropriate areas that you wish to work on. Of course, I am here to help you by what I wrote in this book and I am also available for phone coaching whenever you wish to get started, but in case you decide to hire a personal trainer or other professional to work with your goals "live", here are some things for you to consider in your search for the right fit. Although these tips are specifically geared towards a fitness trainer (since many of you are looking to improve your fitness) several of these points can be used to assess the credentials and personality of any professional you choose to work with.

In my 20 years as a personal trainer I have worked with a lot of individuals and have developed routines that were specifically tailored to each one of them. The ground rules for any of these clients were to develop programming that was safe, and with content built specifically for their body limitations, fitness level, and interests. I spent several years educating and certifying new trainers and tried to instill these same important concepts into them before issuing a diploma. Some trainers get it, others do not.

No matter what certification a trainer holds, if they are from any of the major players in the industry, they all have relatively the same code of ethics in the training manual.

Some key areas include: Responsibility to the public and responsibility to the profession. Trainers should be supplying services in a competent and legal manner within his/her scope of practice.

The services should be provided in a competent, skilled, and passionate manner utilizing *best practice* and always putting safety first. The trainer should maintain high professional standards and continue to educate him/herself in order to maintain the knowledge, skills, and abilities set forth by the certifying agency.

There are several questions you should be asking every potential trainer you might work with in order to find a *professional* who is the perfect fit for you! Here are some of the general questions you should be asking to determine if they are the right fit before purchasing a bundle of sessions.

Question 1: Which organization are they certified by and how long have they been training? The top three certifications for Personal Training are from the ACSM, NSCA, and ACE. There are certainly other organizations that can provide a great certification, but these three are the crème-de-la crème, with the American College of Sports Medicine being number one.

The certifying organization certainly does not dictate exclusively how good of a trainer they will be, but it can tell you the caliber of their training and expertise. Be careful if you find a trainer who gives you the name of some two-bit web-based organization that no one has ever heard of.

Question 2: What is this trainer's specialty?

Personal trainers should be able to work with a variety of individuals at any fitness level; the basic training principles remain the same, but many trainers find a niche market either by happenstance or because of specialty training that they have received.

Find out if the trainer specializes in working with older adults, newbies, college athlete, or serious weight lifters. This will give you a good indication if this trainer is right for you and will meet your needs.

Question 3: What is their fitness philosophy; how do they elicit change in their clients? Ask for a sample plan; what does a typical workout consist of for a beginner, intermediate, or advanced client? These should all be organized a little differently and have tactics in mind that challenge a person at each stage.

This can either be shown to you in print, or a simple verbal description of how they would design a basic workout for your preferred interests and skill level can suffice.

If you are a beginner, one thing to listen for is that they are designing an <u>uncomplicated</u> workout that does not require too much thinking or know-how. (Your initial 2 weeks of weight training should not consist of five different routines.) Also, if you find someone who uses the same routine for everyone, this does not work either; go elsewhere.

Question 4: Do they have any experience with behavior change theories? Personal training is not just about putting you through the paces of a great cardio and weight routine, it is also about learning why the clients either do or don't make lasting changes.

This all starts with basic behavior theory; the most prevalent one used is the Stages of Change model, which is taught in most renowned personal training courses and the one discussed in this book. The trainer should have a basic knowledge of health behavior theory in order to identify how to best elicit change and how to counsel you when you get stuck. If a trainer has no idea what behavior theory is, you may want to keep looking.

Question 5: What feeling do you get when you are speaking with them? Do you click? One of the best indicators you can use when searching for a trainer is your gut! What is your overall feeling when you are first introduced to this person? Are they welcoming, engaging, personable? Whatever qualities you look for in the people you hang around with should be the same that you look for in your trainer. After all, you may very well be spending several hours a week with this person, so you want to enjoy that time! Don't be afraid to discuss the elephant in the room. If your personalities are not a match, just say so and ask if he/she can recommend another trainer that might be better suited for you. Any good trainer should also be able to sense if there is a match or not and should be the first one to recommend the right fit for you.

Question 6: What is their fee and availability? If all of the other parameters fall into place, then the only things left to discuss are "how much" and "when can we start". Fees vary from region to region, but for the most part you can expect to pay between $40.00 and $80.00 per session with a well-qualified trainer.

The more experienced and educated the trainer is, the more you can expect to pay, unless they work in a facility with a fixed rate. Make sure that your schedules jive and that this person has the availability you seek. The next step is to schedule that first session and get started on your path to a brand new you!

Now, while all of these fantastic changes are taking place and you are becoming the "brand new you", remember to give yourself a pat on the back for a job well done! Whether you have completed your Weekly Goals, met your 3-Month Goal, did well with training sessions, or reduced the cigarettes that you smoke, it is important to reward yourself for these achievements! One of the most basic concepts that people forget to integrate into their wellness journey is the reward system.

Whether you desire intrinsic rewards (something on the inside that other people don't necessarily see such as taking time to read a book) or extrinsic (something on the outside that others can see such as a party given in your honor, or a new wardrobe) everyone needs some sort of reward to continue to feel successful in their efforts. After all, if your goal was so important to achieve, why wouldn't you acknowledge and reward the fact that you achieved it? By rewarding yourself, you learn to associate fun and positivity with your accomplishments, and this makes it much more exciting as you continue on your journey towards success and maintain your new habits. When was the last time you bought yourself flowers for a job well done or went to get a pedicure for attaining your goals for the week? It has probably been too long! You need to continue to reward yourself at certain increments of time so that you can continue to stay motivated and strengthen your resolve within the maintenance stage. Likely, no one else is going to do it for you, so you need to take control and do it for yourself! Just make sure it is a non-food reward, since most of you reading this book are seeking some amount of weight loss for your wellness journey. Having food rewards sends the wrong message. "Wow, I lost 2 pounds so now I can have a hot fudge sundae!" Not really.

- Speaking of food, we need to keep in mind the "everything in moderation" philosophy and not put treats into any "off limits" category. Having treats every once in a while when implementing heathy nutrition habits *most* of the time is what is normal; so your hot fudge sundae is simply part of your *normal* wellness plan, not something special to give yourself as a reward for reaching your goals.

Here are some ideas of rewards that you can give yourself for achieving your Weekly Goals, 3-Month Goal, your Wellness Vision, or any other milestone that is important to you. Perhaps you want to keep your rewards smaller during the week and have bigger rewards for the larger milestones. The choice is yours; the point is to have fun and give yourself awareness for all the hard work you have put forth! Your rewards give you a deeper meaning for what you are working so hard on! Many of these ideas my clients have actually used and have had great success. Please try some of them yourself.

1. Stash cash! Try saving $1.00-$5.00 for every pound lost, ounce of water you drink, or

cigarette you did not smoke each week. Whatever you wish! Those dollars add up and can be used to buy yourself something nice or put towards the monthly bills!

2. Give yourself a spa day. Have a manicure or pedicure, get your hair cut or styled differently, get a professional makeup application. Get a massage.

3. Give 30 minutes or more to yourself to do whatever you want!

4. Buy or pick a beautiful bouquet of flowers.

5. Go to a movie with a friend or by yourself, just skip the junk at the concession stand!

6. Redecorate a room in your house or move the furniture around to create a fresh space.

7. Buy tickets to a special concert or sporting event that you normally would not attend;

remember, this is a special occasion!

8. Light some candles and take a long bubble bath. Add some soft music and just relax.

9. Buy a new book that you have wanted to read, then take time to read it!

10. Frame a "certificate of accomplishment" that you create yourself and hang it for all to see.

11. Have a party in your honor and make a formal announcement of your accomplishment.

12. Buy yourself a new piece of jewelry or other wardrobe items. (It is especially important to buy new clothes that fit your new body if you are losing weight. Don't wait until you have lost "all" the weight; you need to have clothes that fit during the process to make you look and feel amazing at whatever size you are!)

13. Take a day off of work.

14. Plan a trip that you have always wanted to take.

This gives you an idea of where to start. I trust that you will think of more ways that you can reward yourself and give merit to your accomplishments. Enjoy yourself during the process of change as you work through your goals towards the Wellness Vision that you have created for yourself. Remember, as Arthur Ashe once said "Success is a journey, not a destination". So let's celebrate our success as we journey on!

- Here is your last stop! Take a moment to make a list of rewards that you would like to give yourself when you achieve both small and larger goals. This is the fun part! Dream big!

So friends, now it is time for you to make a choice to start on your own journey towards optimal wellness, or perhaps you have already begun the process while reading this book and are beginning to maintain your new-found habits! I truly hope that you can use the tools outlined in these pages to make lasting change once and for all. The keys to your success are recognizing what you want, creating goals, and keeping things interesting while maintaining your habits. Continually reinforce that positive self-talk to help motivate and reinforce your hopes and dreams of the future, and reward yourself when your dreams start to turn into reality because of the good choices you are making. Now is your time to achieve lifetime behavior change; enjoy the process every step of the way. Remember, you CAN do it, and I know you will! Good luck on your journey!

Fitness Resources

Some great fitness-related resources are listed here. Take some time to peruse each website to see what tools and strategies might work for you. Many offer free downloads, pamphlets, fitness calculators, recipes, and more! The first four sites are those that I am affiliated with for those of you who may want to dig a little deeper and do some one-on-one coaching with the author herself, or simply read some of my articles!

www.facebook.com/minutemoves (This page is my one-stop-shop for my Minute Moves videos, motivational messages, coaching call sign up, and a way to contact me directly. Please "like" the page and get started with the workouts!)

www.fitmo.com (Direct from Amsterdam is a new and innovative way to personal train with me; on your mobile device or computer! Log on and check out the coaches page to find me and sign up for the motivation you deserve!)

www.bootcamphub.com (This fee-based online gym has it all, including me and 15 other coaches that will lead you through daily <u>live</u> exercise videos full of motivation and support! We offer nutritional support, specialty courses, phone coaching, live and online retreats, and much more! You will love the personal and friendly approach at Boot Camp Hub, so please try us out today!)

www.askthetrainer.com (A fitness enthusiasts resource full of articles from yours truly, as well as many other qualified professionals that explain the dos and don'ts of fitness, as well as tricks of the trade. Options of asking personal training questions as well as having a total fitness workup are offered by me on the site; fees apply.)

Fitness calculators: These calculators will help you figure out your target heart rate, BMR, calorie intake, suggested weight loss, and more!

www.active.com/fitness/calculators/bodyfat

http://www.active.com/fitness/calculators/heartrate

http://www.bmi-calculator.net/bmr-calculator/

Other online resources for tips, ideas, and motivation!

www.myfitnesspal.com (This is a great resource and an excellent way to track your food and water intake and daily exercise. The food journaling is made easy as the site has thousands of entries from your brand-name foods to local grocery store brands. It also has a recipe option where you can input the amounts and types of food in your recipe and it will calculate the calories for you! There are also several weight loss and calorie calculators as well.)

www.choosemyplate.gov (This is your one-stop-shop for nutrition and fitness guidelines, support, ideas, and tools! Log on to research what foods should be on your plate, how much and what type of exercise you should be getting, and printable grids and checklists to keep you on track. Peruse the "tools" tab to see the many options offered, including **Supertracker** where you can get personalized daily e-mail support and calculators to help you on your fitness journey!)

www.cdc.gov (The CDC is not just about disease prevention; they have a wide array of health topics on their site under the "Healthy Living" tab. Check out the food safety topics, obesity issues, as well as smoking cessation!)

www.diabetes.org (Along with all the information one needs about Type 1 and Type 2 diabetes, this website offers a host of other benefits. Check out the "Food and Fitness" tab to get information about different diets like gluten free and vegetarian, but also peruse a ton of recipes that are quick, easy, and full of nutrients. There is even a holiday meal planning guide.)

www.americanheart.org (Not only will you find information and education about heart disease, but there is also a "Healthy Living" tab that has oodles of information about healthy eating, physical activity, healthy kids, stress reduction, smoking cessation, and even workplace health!)

Bibliography

ACSM's Resources for the Personal Trainer. (2004).
ACSM: Lippincott Williams & Wilkins. Philadelphia.
[This resource is a must have for all fitness trainers.
The manual expertly discusses the foundations of
strength training and conditioning and devotes
chapters to specifics of training, tissues and systems
involved, equipment, and different types of resistance
training. Various exercise physiology information
related to cardiovascular and muscle-toning exercises
was taken from this resource.]

Moore, M. & Tschannen-Moran, B. (2010).

WellCoaches Coaching Psychology Manual. Chap 8.

Philadelphia: Lippincott Williams & Wilkins. [In this

professional certification manual, the psychology

behind behavior change is discussed in order to build

a better foundation for professionals in the health and

wellness coaching field. They teach evidence-based

coaching psychology within the 12-chapters with a

focus on how to understand a client and then how to

initiate change with goal-setting and motivational

strategies. I referred to the Wellness Vision, 3-Month

Goal, and Weekly Goals within my book; all of which

comes from my WellCoaches training and this

manual.]

Sharma & Romas. Theoretical Foundations of Health
Education and Health Promotion. P71.2008:Jones and
Bartlett. Bartlett [In this book, the authors' review the
foundations of health education and promotion by
explaining in detail the various models and theories
used for behavior change. As it is explained,
approaches taken depend on the needs of the
individual and different models should be used
depending on this. The final few chapters also discuss
the social aspects of behavior change and how health
innovations are marketed and accepted by the public.
Specifics of the Health Belief Model as well as the
Stages of Change model were found in this book.]

www.ingramcontent.com/pod-product-compliance
Lightning Source LLC
Chambersburg PA
CBHW070146290526

45789CB00002B/657